Low Cholesterol Food List

Increase Hdl and Lower Ldl Level Naturally with Eating and Diet

By: Frederic Dawson

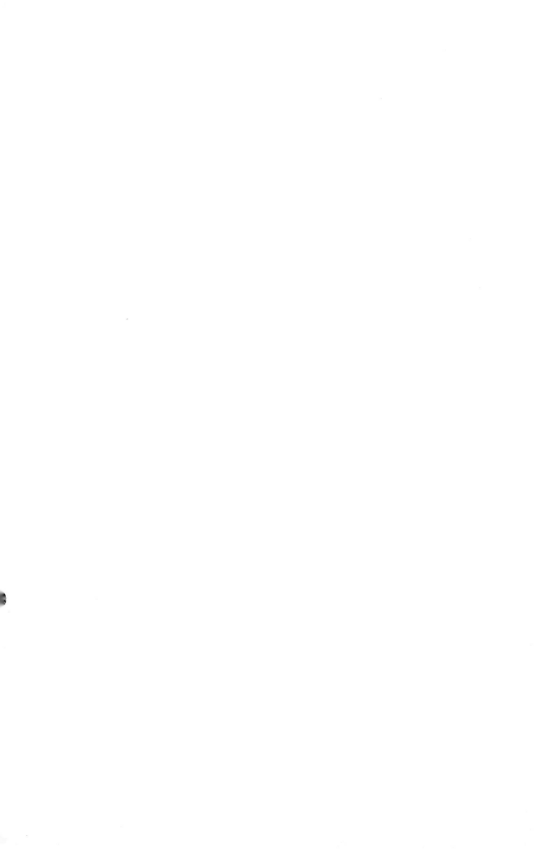

Copyrights:

Disclaimer :

The information contained in this book is for information only, it is not replacing professional consultation about cholesterol, and it is not intended to give any medical advice. The nutritional information about food contents is extracted from the official USDA nutrition database available for the public.

Please feel free to email us at latcarl3@gmail.com for any remark.

About this book :

This book is a practical guide about cholesterol diet, nutrition, and lifestyle. The guide is made up of three major parts:

Part 1:

In part 1 of this book, you will find a condensed guide that covers nutrition and lifestyle, you will discover practical advice, and information to keep your cholesterol level in the right range by increasing the good cholesterol level (HDL), and decreasing the bad cholesterol level (LDL) in the blood.

Part 2:

You will find a huge list of more than 1100 foods with their cholesterol level, this list will help you to consume the right foods and avoid the bad ones for your health.

Part 3:

Is a Safe grocery list of foods that are low in cholesterol, use this list to do your groceries with no worry .

Table of Contents

I. What is cholesterol ? *2*

II. What cholesterol is good, and what cholesterol is bad?..*3*

III. What cholesterol level is normal, good, and bad *5*

IV. What cholesterol level requires medication *7*

V. Why your cholesterol level is high? *8*

VI. Cholesterol symptoms *12*

VII. Can cholesterol be cured completely? *14*

VIII. The best ways to reduce cholesterol..........................*16*

IX. The Comprehensive Cholesterol food list *20*

I. What is cholesterol ?

Cholesterol is a type of fat (waxy-like) substance that the human body produces naturally. Cholesterol is one of the most important substances that help cells to compose vitamin D, hormones (including testosterone and estrogen), and necessary substances for food digestion.

80% of the cholesterol you need is produced by your body, and only 20% comes from the foods you eat. The cholesterol is made by your liver and your intestines, then the body covers the cholesterol particles with proteins to ease their circulation in the bloodstream throughout the body. when the cholesterol particles by proteins, then we get two types of cholesterol:

1. The LDL: low-density lipoprotein (bad cholesterol)

2. The HDL: high-density lipoprotein (good Cholesterol)

II. What cholesterol is good, and what cholesterol is bad?

II. 1 Bad cholesterol:

As stated before, there are two types of cholesterol:

1. The LDL: low-density lipoprotein (bad cholesterol)

2. The HDL: high-density lipoprotein (good Cholesterol)

LDL is called "bad cholesterol" because it increases the risk of heart attacks and other blood pressure diseases. If the LDL concentration in the blood is too high, the body can't dissolve it, so it builds up on the walls of blood vessels, over time, these blood vessels narrow from the inside causing blood circulation problems from the heart to other organs and vice-versa.

to lower the LDL, you should:

- Avoid foods high in saturated

- Avoid foods that are high in sodium

- Avoid sugar-added food

- Eat foods naturally high in fiber (visit our website: www.diabetes2.club to get for free the printable version of our comprehensive high-fiber food list)

- Exercise regularly

- Maintain a healthy weight

- Stop smoking.

II.2 good cholesterol :

HDL is called the "Good cholesterol" because it plays a major role in preventing heart attacks and blood vessel diseases, it removes the LDL by transporting it back to the liver to be reprocessed, it maintains the walls of blood vessels, and maintains the stability of every cell in the body.

a good level of HDL in the body should not be less than 40 mg/dl, an optimal value should be greater than 60 mg/dl.

There are several ways to increase the concentration of HDL in the body, including:

- Exercise regularly at least for 30 min 4 times a week (at least)

- Maintain a healthy weight, and stop smoking

III. What cholesterol level is normal, good, and bad

The measure of cholesterol is made via cholesterol blood test, this test measures the two types of cholesterol LDL and HDL, and the unit of measure is the mg/dl (milligrams per deciliter).

it's worth mentioning that cholesterol is a silent disease, it has (almost) no symptoms. It is recommended to do cholesterol checking on a regular way according to your sex, age, and health conditions, here are some guidelines:

For men aged under 45: Cholesterol test every 5 years

For men aged between 45 to 65: every 2 years

For Women aged under 55: Cholesterol test every 5 years

For women aged between 55 to 65: every 2 years

for people with specific conditions like diabetes, blood pressure,…cholesterol checking should be conducted every year.

So what is a normal, good, and bad cholesterol value?

According to the CDC (US centers for diseases control and prevention):

- **LDL (bad cholesterol)** should be **Less than 100 mg/dL**
- **HDL (good cholesterol)** should be **Greater than or equal to 60 mg/dL**
- **Triglycerides** should be less than **150 mg/dL**
- and finally, **Total cholesterol** should be **Less than 200 mg/dL**

Triglycerides are a type of fats that your body extracts from fatty foods (like oil, and butter...), they are also produced from extra calories that your body does not need right away. The measuring of triglycerides during a cholesterol check can predict the occurrence of stroke attacks and prevent them.

IV. What cholesterol level requires medication

Cholesterol level is qualified as dangerous when the LDL value is greater than 16O mg/dl, or when the HDL is lower than 40 mg/dl, or when the total cholesterol value is greater than 240 mg/dl, at this point, your doctor may prescribe some medication to bring back the cholesterol value to its normal range, these medicines or drugs bloc some substances that the body uses to compose cholesterol.

Dangerous cholesterol values may increase the risk of heart attacks, and strokes, this risk may be accelerated by a non-healthy lifestyle, heredity, and other factors, so it is always a wise decision to see a doctor when you have high cholesterol readings.

Are cholesterol drugs bad for you?

The drugs used to adjust cholesterol levels are called "Statins", they also decrease the risk of strokes and heart attacks. Being on Statins or not is a decision that only your doctor can make based on your risk factors, cholesterol level, overall health, and family history. finally, statins have some small side effects like headaches, nausea, and muscle pain, however, these symptoms disappear in most cases after a certain time, especially if you maintain a healthy lifestyle.

V. Why your cholesterol level is high?

There are several factors that lead to high and unhealthy cholesterol levels, these factors are mainly:
bad nutrition: the consumption of too much-saturated fats, and a diet poor in fibers.

- **Unhealthy lifestyle:** including lack of activity, drinking too much coffee, and stress

- **Age:** being over 40 is also a risk factor

- **Smoking**: the substances present in the cigarettes block the production of HDL, and as we know, the HDL is

Cholesterol with keto diet: is it safe?

The keto diet consists of reducing carbs consumption (less than 60 g a day), and increasing proteins and fats part, in this scenario, people with high cholesterol LDL are advisable to not start a keto diet as it may increase even more the LDL concentration in the blood, putting more stress on kidneys and heart.

Sometimes keto diet may be beneficial for some high cholesterol patients, in this case, it should be strictly under the supervision of a doctor .

responsible for decreasing the LDL, so when HDL is blocked, the LDL concentration increases in the blood, which may lead to heart attacks and strokes.

- **Pregnancy:** during pregnancy you may have high cholesterol, but this is temporary during the third trimester, however, if you already have cholesterol, then you need to see your doctor to track your cholesterol level each month.

- **Heredity**: people with a cholesterol history in the family should watch closely their cholesterol level, especially after the 40s.

- **Diabetes**: diabetics (especially type 2) with poor sugar level control tend to have high cholesterol levels more than other people, this condition is called: dyslipidemia. In this case, the person should be treated for both conditions: Cholesterol and diabetes.

Are you a type 2 diabetic?

then controlling your blood sugar level should be your priority along with consuming non-starchy food. We have produced printable food lists and nutrition guides that will help you to maintain an optimal blood sugar level.

please visit us at :

www.diabetes2.club

- **High-crabs diet**

- **Alcohol:** alcohol is also processed by the liver as well as cholesterol, too much alcohol consumption may alter your liver function and causes cholesterol level to increase drastically.

- **Kidney problems**

VI. Cholesterol symptoms

As we mentioned before in this book, cholesterol is a silent disease and needs blood tests to confirm its presence, however, the human body let out some signs and symptoms when the bad cholesterol (LDL) level is too high in the blood, or when the good cholesterol (HDL) level is too low.

The following symptoms could be taken as warning signs, but, these symptoms are not related directly to cholesterol rather than to its complications like heart problems, and blood vessels issue. If you express any one of these signs, then make an appointment with your doctor as soon as you could.

Warning symptoms:

- Angina
- breath shortness.
- chest pain.

Cholesterol and inflammation

The cholesterol itself doesn't cause inflammation, however, a high LDL cholesterol level in the blood reduces the ability of the body to fight against inflammation.

NB: The HDL cholesterol has an anti-inflammatory function, so when the LDL is low and the HDL is high, the inflammation retreats.

- extreme fatigue.
- nausea.
- numbness or coldness in your hands and legs.
- pain in jaw
- pain in the neck

Will cholesterol cause dizziness?

Too much cholesterol in the blood may lead to plaque formation, these plaques are basically a type of fats that cover the interior walls of blood vessels causing a partial blockage of the blood flow from and to the heart, this condition may lead to dizziness that high cholesterol patients suffer from.

VII. Can cholesterol be cured completely?

Will your cholesterol go away? the short and final answer to this question is YES. Period! cholesterol is a condition that can be cured by making some changes in lifestyle, nutrition, and sometimes taking medication if needed.

How long does it take to get rid of cholesterol?

Bringing cholesterol values back to their normal range may take some time, it can take from 8 to 12 weeks if the right lifestyle is adopted, and sometimes it may take months, but it really varies from one person to another, however, if the cholesterol level hasn't dropped for more than three months, the doctor may prescribe some medicines to boost the process.

It's advisable to discuss with your doctor the right plan to reduce your cholesterol, your doctor will then consider your overall health condition, your family history, and your lifestyle to give you a cholesterol-reducing plan. in the next chapter, you will find some general (and practical) guidelines on how to reduce cholesterol.

You can visit our website : www.diabetes2.club, to get a cholesterol-reducing planner to help you in this process

VIII. The best ways to reduce cholesterol

Reducing cholesterol is easier than you think, all you need is to tweak a little bit your lifestyle, eat the right nutrition, and avoid smoking and drinking alchohol.

the second part of this book is all about eating the right food and avoiding the bad ones, but, let us give you some quick changes to start with:

- **Avoid trans fats**: this means avoiding as much as possible pastries, cookies, fast foods, margarine…

- **Consume more monosaturated fats:** this means consuming more olives and olive oil, avocado, nuts, nuts butter and nuts oil, canola oil…

- **Consume Omega-3 rich foods**: this means consuming more salmon, tuna, shellfish, and mackerel

- **Eat soluble fibers** like oatmeal, beans, chickpeas, flaxseeds,

- **Eat more fruits and vegetables**

Cholesterol-lowering foods:

There are some foods that contribute to lowering LDL cholesterol, here are some of these foods:

- *Oats*
- oat bran
- *Barley*
- *whole grains*
- *Beans*
- *Eggplant*
- *Okra*
- *Walnuts*
- peanuts
- almonds
- canola oil
- sunflower oil
- safflower oil
- *Apples,*
- *grapes,*
- *strawberries,*
- *citrus fruits*
- orange juice
- chocolate
- granola bars
- soybeans
- soy milk
- tofu
- fatty fish
- psyllium (fiber supplement)

Besides the right nutrition, exercising is the second most important factor to lower LDL cholesterol, a 30 min walk every two days is what experts recommend to lower cholesterol.

To lower LDL cholesterol and increase the HDL, you should also maintain a healthy weight. Every pound of excess weight is responsible for producing extra mg of cholesterol each day, and vice-versa, each excess pound of weight lost, is a significant decrease in the cholesterol level.

We advise working closely with your doctor to develop a customized weight loss plan for you along with a suitable meal plan.

Cholesterol supplements:

There are several supplements that have a lowering power over cholesterol, the most know are the **sterols and the stanols**.

these two supplements are extracted from plants and have been proved to lower cholesterol.

Before taking any of these supplements, talk to your doctor.

NB : *The USDA has a cooking guide to preparing healthy food on a budget for high cholesterol people, you can get* *it for free on the USDA website, or you can visit www.diabetes2.club to get it directly.*

IX. The Comprehensive Cholesterol food list

This is the most comprehensive food list about cholesterol, it list covers (almost) all types of foods including:

- Vegetables
- Fruits
- Nuts and seeds
- Grains and pasta
- Meat
- Fish
- Beverages
- Baked foods
- Beans and lentils
- Dairy and egg products
- Snacks, and more…

The list is organized following the alphabet order. There are four types of food categories according to the cholesterol concentration:

- Safe: the food has ZERO cholesterol
- Low in cholesterol
- Medium in cholesterol
- High in cholesterol
- Very high in cholesterol

Generally speaking, you should avoid "high" and "very high cholesterol" foods, however, if you have other medical conditions like diabetes or blood pressure, then avoid also "medium in cholesterol" foods.

If you want a specific list of foods that are only "Safe" and "Low in cholesterol", then check the last ten pages of this book. Use this list to do your grocery.

Note 1 :

we have removed alcoholic beverages from the list as you should avoid them to control your cholesterol.

Note 2:

In order to qualify the foods in this list, we use the method of the %DV.

The %DV is the percentage of the cholesterol in a food compared to the recommended daily cholesterol value which is 300 mg per serving.

This is how the %DV is calculated:

(the amount of the cholesterol in a food per servin/300) x 100

- The foods that have a %DV less than 5% are qualified as low cholesterol

- If the %DV is between 5% and 20%, then the food is medium in cholesterol

- If the %DV is between 20% and 100%, the the food is high in cholesterl

- Foods that have a %DV higher than 100%, are qualified as very high in cholesterol

Food Name	Cholesterol (mg)	Cholesterol DV	Comment
Amaranth	0	0%	SAFE (No Cholesterol)
Artichokes	0	0%	SAFE (No Cholesterol)
Atlantic Cod	55	18%	Medium In Cholesterol
Atlantic Perch	63	21%	High in Cholesterol
Beet Greens	0	0%	SAFE (No Cholesterol)
Beets	0	0%	SAFE (No Cholesterol)
Blackeyed Peas	0	0%	SAFE (No Cholesterol)
Blue Mussels	56	19%	Medium In Cholesterol
Broadbeans	0	0%	SAFE (No Cholesterol)
Broccoli Raab	0	0%	SAFE (No Cholesterol)
Brown Rice	0	0%	SAFE (No Cholesterol)
Bulgur	0	0%	SAFE (No Cholesterol)
Burdock Root	0	0%	SAFE (No Cholesterol)
Butternut Squash	0	0%	SAFE (No Cholesterol)
Cabbage	0	0%	SAFE (No Cholesterol)
Carrots	0	0%	SAFE (No Cholesterol)
Catfish	72	24%	High in Cholesterol
Catjang Beans	0	0%	SAFE (No Cholesterol)
Cauliflower	0	0%	SAFE (No Cholesterol)
Celeriac	0	0%	SAFE (No Cholesterol)
Celery	0	0%	SAFE (No Cholesterol)
Chayote	0	0%	SAFE (No Cholesterol)
Chicken Breast	73	24%	High in Cholesterol
Chinese Broccoli	0	0%	SAFE (No Cholesterol)
Chrysanthemum	0	0%	SAFE (No Cholesterol)
Clams	67	22%	High in Cholesterol
Cod	61	20%	High in Cholesterol
Coho Salmon (Farmed)	63	21%	High in Cholesterol
Coho Salmon (Wild Moist F	57	19%	Medium In Cholesterol
Coho Salmon (Wild)	55	18%	Medium In Cholesterol
Collards	0	0%	SAFE (No Cholesterol)

Food Name	Cholesterol (mg)	Cholesterol DV	Comment
Couscous	0	0%	SAFE (No Cholesterol)
Crayfish	137	46%	High in Cholesterol
Crookneck Summer Squash	0	0%	SAFE (No Cholesterol)
Cuttlefish	224	75%	High in Cholesterol
Dandelion Greens	0	0%	SAFE (No Cholesterol)
Deer Tenderloin	88	29%	High in Cholesterol
Dungeness Crab	76	25%	High in Cholesterol
Eggplant	0	0%	SAFE (No Cholesterol)
Escarole	0	0%	SAFE (No Cholesterol)
Green Cauliflower	0	0%	SAFE (No Cholesterol)
Green Peas	0	0%	SAFE (No Cholesterol)
Kale	0	0%	SAFE (No Cholesterol)
Leeks	0	0%	SAFE (No Cholesterol)
Lentil Sprouts	0	0%	SAFE (No Cholesterol)
Lima Beans	0	0%	SAFE (No Cholesterol)
Lingcod	67	22%	High in Cholesterol
Lotus Root	0	0%	SAFE (No Cholesterol)
Mahimahi	94	31%	High in Cholesterol
Malabar Spinach	0	0%	SAFE (No Cholesterol)
Millet	0	0%	SAFE (No Cholesterol)
Mustard Greens	0	0%	SAFE (No Cholesterol)
Oat Bran	0	0%	SAFE (No Cholesterol)
Oatmeal	0	0%	SAFE (No Cholesterol)
Okra	0	0%	SAFE (No Cholesterol)
Onions	0	0%	SAFE (No Cholesterol)
Orange Roughy	80	27%	High in Cholesterol
Pacific Cod	57	19%	Medium In Cholesterol
Pacific Herring	99	33%	High in Cholesterol
Pacific Oysters	100	33%	High in Cholesterol
Parsnips	0	0%	SAFE (No Cholesterol)
Pasta (Unenriched)	0	0%	SAFE (No Cholesterol)
Peanuts	0	0%	SAFE (No Cholesterol)
Pollock	91	30%	High in Cholesterol

Food Name	Cholesterol (mg)	Cholesterol DV	Comment
Pompano	64	21%	High in Cholesterol
Pumpkin	0	0%	SAFE (No Cholesterol)
Pumpkin Flowers	0	0%	SAFE (No Cholesterol)
Purslane	0	0%	SAFE (No Cholesterol)
Red Cabbage	0	0%	SAFE (No Cholesterol)
Red Kidney Beans	0	0%	SAFE (No Cholesterol)
Rutabagas (Neeps Swedes)	0	0%	SAFE (No Cholesterol)
Sablefish	63	21%	High in Cholesterol
Savoy Cabbage	0	0%	SAFE (No Cholesterol)
Scallop Squash	0	0%	SAFE (No Cholesterol)
Scallops	24	8%	Medium In Cholesterol
Sea Bass	53	18%	Medium In Cholesterol
Sesame Butter (Tahini)	0	0%	SAFE (No Cholesterol)
Shrimp	211	70%	High in Cholesterol
Skipjack	60	20%	Medium In Cholesterol
Smelt	90	30%	High in Cholesterol
Snapper	47	16%	Medium In Cholesterol
Snow Peas	0	0%	SAFE (No Cholesterol)
Spinach	0	0%	SAFE (No Cholesterol)
Taro	0	0%	SAFE (No Cholesterol)
Teff	0	0%	SAFE (No Cholesterol)
Tilapia	57	19%	Medium In Cholesterol
Tilefish	64	21%	High in Cholesterol
Tomatoes	0	0%	SAFE (No Cholesterol)
Trout	69	23%	High in Cholesterol
Turbot	62	21%	High in Cholesterol
Turnip Greens	0	0%	SAFE (No Cholesterol)
Turnips	0	0%	SAFE (No Cholesterol)
Walleye Pike	110	37%	High in Cholesterol
Whitefish	77	26%	High in Cholesterol
Whiting	84	28%	High in Cholesterol
Wild Rice	0	0%	SAFE (No Cholesterol)
Winter Squash	0	0%	SAFE (No Cholesterol)

Food Name	Cholesterol (mg)	Cholesterol DV	Comment
Yam	0	0%	SAFE (No Cholesterol)
Yellow Snap Beans	0	0%	SAFE (No Cholesterol)
Yellow Sweet Corn	0	0%	SAFE (No Cholesterol)
Yellowfin Tuna	47	16%	Medium In Cholesterol
Yellowtail	71	24%	High in Cholesterol
Zucchini	0	0%	SAFE (No Cholesterol)
Abalone	94	31%	High in Cholesterol
Acerola Juice	0	0%	SAFE (No Cholesterol)
Acorn Squash	0	0%	SAFE (No Cholesterol)
Acorns	0	0%	SAFE (No Cholesterol)
Adzuki Beans	0	0%	SAFE (No Cholesterol)
Agave	0	0%	SAFE (No Cholesterol)
Alfalfa Sprouts	0	0%	SAFE (No Cholesterol)
Alfredo Sauce	45	15%	Medium In Cholesterol
Almond Butter	0	0%	SAFE (No Cholesterol)
Almond Chicken	57	19%	Medium In Cholesterol
Almond Joy Candy Bar	4	1%	Low in Cholesterol
Almond Milk Unsweetened	0	0%	SAFE (No Cholesterol)
Almond Oil	0	0%	SAFE (No Cholesterol)
Almond Paste	0	0%	SAFE (No Cholesterol)
Almonds	0	0%	SAFE (No Cholesterol)
Aloe Vera Juice Drink Fortifi	0	0%	SAFE (No Cholesterol)
Alpen	0	0%	SAFE (No Cholesterol)
Amaranth Grain Un	0	0%	SAFE (No Cholesterol)
Ambrosia	0	0%	SAFE (No Cholesterol)
American Cheese	98	33%	High in Cholesterol
Anchovies	60	20%	Medium In Cholesterol
Anise Seeds	0	0%	SAFE (No Cholesterol)
Apple Juice	0	0%	SAFE (No Cholesterol)
Apples	0	0%	SAFE (No Cholesterol)
Applesauce Canned or Unsw	0	0%	SAFE (No Cholesterol)
Apricots	0	0%	SAFE (No Cholesterol)
Archway Home Style Cookie	0	0%	SAFE (No Cholesterol)

Food Name	Cholesterol (mg)	Cholesterol DV	Comment
Arrowhead	0	0%	SAFE (No Cholesterol)
Arrowroot	0	0%	SAFE (No Cholesterol)
Artichokes	3	1%	Low in Cholesterol
Arugula	0	0%	SAFE (No Cholesterol)
Asian Pears	0	0%	SAFE (No Cholesterol)
Asparagus	0	0%	SAFE (No Cholesterol)
Atlantic Herring	77	26%	High in Cholesterol
Atlantic Mackerel	75	25%	High in Cholesterol
Avocado Oil	0	0%	SAFE (No Cholesterol)
Avocados	0	0%	SAFE (No Cholesterol)
Baby Carrots	0	0%	SAFE (No Cholesterol)
Baby Ruth	0	0%	SAFE (No Cholesterol)
Bacon	66	22%	High in Cholesterol
Bacon And Beef Sticks	102	34%	High in Cholesterol
Bagel	0	0%	SAFE (No Cholesterol)
Baklava	45	15%	Medium In Cholesterol
Balsamic Vinegar	0	0%	SAFE (No Cholesterol)
Bamboo Shoots	0	0%	SAFE (No Cholesterol)
Bananas	0	0%	SAFE (No Cholesterol)
Barbecue Sauce	0	0%	SAFE (No Cholesterol)
Bartlett Pears	0	0%	SAFE (No Cholesterol)
Basbousa	3	1%	Low in Cholesterol
Basil	0	0%	SAFE (No Cholesterol)
Bay Leaves	0	0%	SAFE (No Cholesterol)
Bean Cake	0	0%	SAFE (No Cholesterol)
Bean Chips	0	0%	SAFE (No Cholesterol)
Beans Yellow Mature Seeds	0	0%	SAFE (No Cholesterol)
Bear	98	33%	High in Cholesterol
Beaver	117	39%	High in Cholesterol
Beet Greens	0	0%	SAFE (No Cholesterol)
Beets	0	0%	SAFE (No Cholesterol)
Biryani With Chicken	25	8%	Medium In Cholesterol
Biryani With Meat	29	10%	Medium In Cholesterol

Food Name	Cholesterol (mg)	Cholesterol DV	Comment
Biryani With Vegetables	8	3%	Low in Cholesterol
Biscuit Cheese	12	4%	Low in Cholesterol
Bison	82	27%	High in Cholesterol
Bitter Melon	0	0%	SAFE (No Cholesterol)
Black Beans	0	0%	SAFE (No Cholesterol)
Black Tea (Brewed)	0	0%	SAFE (No Cholesterol)
Black-Eyed Peas (Cowpeas)	0	0%	SAFE (No Cholesterol)
Blackberries	0	0%	SAFE (No Cholesterol)
Blintz Cheese-Filled	85	28%	High in Cholesterol
Blintz Fruit-Filled	66	22%	High in Cholesterol
Blood Sausage	120	40%	High in Cholesterol
Blue Cheese	75	25%	High in Cholesterol
Blue Crab	97	32%	High in Cholesterol
Blueberries	0	0%	SAFE (No Cholesterol)
Bluefin Tuna	49	16%	Medium In Cholesterol
Bok Choy	0	0%	SAFE (No Cholesterol)
Borage	0	0%	SAFE (No Cholesterol)
Borscht	5	2%	Low in Cholesterol
Bosc Pear	0	0%	SAFE (No Cholesterol)
Bottled Water	0	0%	SAFE (No Cholesterol)
Boysenberries	0	0%	SAFE (No Cholesterol)
Boysenberries Canned Heavy	0	0%	SAFE (No Cholesterol)
Braised Beef Or Chuck Stew	99	33%	High in Cholesterol
Brazilnuts	0	0%	SAFE (No Cholesterol)
Bread Cheese	10	3%	Low in Cholesterol
Bread Egg	51	17%	Medium In Cholesterol
Bread Fruit	41	14%	Medium In Cholesterol
Bread Italian	0	0%	SAFE (No Cholesterol)
Bread Nut	46	15%	Medium In Cholesterol
Bread Oat Bran	0	0%	SAFE (No Cholesterol)
Bread Oat Bran Toasted	0	0%	SAFE (No Cholesterol)
Bread Oatmeal	0	0%	SAFE (No Cholesterol)
Bread Oatmeal Toasted	0	0%	SAFE (No Cholesterol)

Food Name	Cholesterol (mg)	Cholesterol DV	Comment
Bread Onion	3	1%	Low in Cholesterol
Bread Onion Toasted	4	1%	Low in Cholesterol
Bread Potato	0	0%	SAFE (No Cholesterol)
Bread Potato Toasted	0	0%	SAFE (No Cholesterol)
Bread Soy	4	1%	Low in Cholesterol
Breast Milk (Human)	14	5%	Low in Cholesterol
Brick Cheese	94	31%	High in Cholesterol
Brioche	158	53%	High in Cholesterol
Broccoli	0	0%	SAFE (No Cholesterol)
Brown Rice	0	0%	SAFE (No Cholesterol)
Brunswick Stew	37	12%	Medium In Cholesterol
Bruschetta	0	0%	SAFE (No Cholesterol)
Brussels Sprouts	0	0%	SAFE (No Cholesterol)
Burdock Root	0	0%	SAFE (No Cholesterol)
Burrito With Beans	2	1%	Low in Cholesterol
Burrito With Meat	41	14%	Medium In Cholesterol
Butter Croissants	67	22%	High in Cholesterol
Butterhead Lettuce	0	0%	SAFE (No Cholesterol)
Buttermilk	11	4%	Low in Cholesterol
Butternut Squash	0	0%	SAFE (No Cholesterol)
Butternuts	0	0%	SAFE (No Cholesterol)
Caay Cheese	93	31%	High in Cholesterol
Caay Seed	0	0%	SAFE (No Cholesterol)
Cabbage	0	0%	SAFE (No Cholesterol)
Cabbage Creamed	3	1%	Low in Cholesterol
Caffeine Free Cola	0	0%	SAFE (No Cholesterol)
Cake Jelly Roll	58	19%	Medium In Cholesterol
Cake Or Cupcake Oatmeal	17	6%	Medium In Cholesterol
California Avocados	0	0%	SAFE (No Cholesterol)
California Grapefruit	0	0%	SAFE (No Cholesterol)
California Red Kidney Bean	0	0%	SAFE (No Cholesterol)
California Valencia Oranges	0	0%	SAFE (No Cholesterol)
Camambert	72	24%	High in Cholesterol

Food Name	Cholesterol (mg)	Cholesterol DV	Comment
Canadian Bacon	48	16%	Medium In Cholesterol
Canadian Bacon (Pan-Fried)	67	22%	High in Cholesterol
Candied Tamarind	0	0%	SAFE (No Cholesterol)
Canned Anchovies	85	28%	High in Cholesterol
Canned Asparagus	0	0%	SAFE (No Cholesterol)
Canned Atlantic Cod	55	18%	Medium In Cholesterol
Canned Baked Beans	0	0%	SAFE (No Cholesterol)
Canned Baked Beans With E	22	7%	Medium In Cholesterol
Canned Blue Crab	97	32%	High in Cholesterol
Canned Chili With Beans	17	6%	Medium In Cholesterol
Canned Clams	50	17%	Medium In Cholesterol
Canned Cranberry Beans	0	0%	SAFE (No Cholesterol)
Canned Eastern Oysters	55	18%	Medium In Cholesterol
Canned Green Beans	0	0%	SAFE (No Cholesterol)
Canned Ham	49	16%	Medium In Cholesterol
Canned Hominy	0	0%	SAFE (No Cholesterol)
Canned Kidney Beans	0	0%	SAFE (No Cholesterol)
Canned Mushrooms	0	0%	SAFE (No Cholesterol)
Canned Navy Beans	0	0%	SAFE (No Cholesterol)
Canned Orange Juice	0	0%	SAFE (No Cholesterol)
Canned Pimentos	0	0%	SAFE (No Cholesterol)
Canned Salmon	79	26%	High in Cholesterol
Canned Sardines	142	47%	High in Cholesterol
Canned Shrimp	252	84%	High in Cholesterol
Canola Oil	0	0%	SAFE (No Cholesterol)
Cantaloupe Melons	0	0%	SAFE (No Cholesterol)
Cantaloupe Nectar	0	0%	SAFE (No Cholesterol)
Capers	0	0%	SAFE (No Cholesterol)
Caramel Candy	7	2%	Low in Cholesterol
Caramel With Nuts	6	2%	Low in Cholesterol
Cardamom	0	0%	SAFE (No Cholesterol)
Carignane	0	0%	SAFE (No Cholesterol)
Carissa	0	0%	SAFE (No Cholesterol)

Food Name	Cholesterol (mg)	Cholesterol DV	Comment
Carp Smoked	103	34%	High in Cholesterol
Carrots	0	0%	SAFE (No Cholesterol)
Casaba Melon	0	0%	SAFE (No Cholesterol)
Cashews	0	0%	SAFE (No Cholesterol)
Cassava	0	0%	SAFE (No Cholesterol)
Catfish Baked Or Broiled Mi	75	25%	High in Cholesterol
Cauliflower	0	0%	SAFE (No Cholesterol)
Cauliflower Pickled	0	0%	SAFE (No Cholesterol)
Cayenne Pepper	0	0%	SAFE (No Cholesterol)
Celeriac	0	0%	SAFE (No Cholesterol)
Celery	0	0%	SAFE (No Cholesterol)
Celery Creamed	3	1%	Low in Cholesterol
Celery Pickled	0	0%	SAFE (No Cholesterol)
Celery Seed	0	0%	SAFE (No Cholesterol)
Celtuce	0	0%	SAFE (No Cholesterol)
Cereal (General Mills 25% L	0	0%	SAFE (No Cholesterol)
Cereal Beverage	0	0%	SAFE (No Cholesterol)
Cereal Granola	0	0%	SAFE (No Cholesterol)
Cereal Muesli	0	0%	SAFE (No Cholesterol)
Cereal Nestum	0	0%	SAFE (No Cholesterol)
Cereal Oat	0	0%	SAFE (No Cholesterol)
Cereal Rice Flakes	0	0%	SAFE (No Cholesterol)
Ceviche	18	6%	Medium In Cholesterol
Chardonnay	0	0%	SAFE (No Cholesterol)
Chayote Fruit	0	0%	SAFE (No Cholesterol)
Cheddar Cheese	99	33%	High in Cholesterol
Cheese Dip	8	3%	Low in Cholesterol
Cheese Fondue	68	23%	High in Cholesterol
Cheese Goat	77	26%	High in Cholesterol
Cheese Ricotta	41	14%	Medium In Cholesterol
Cheese Sauce	8	3%	Low in Cholesterol
Cherries (Sweet)	0	0%	SAFE (No Cholesterol)
Chestnuts	0	0%	SAFE (No Cholesterol)

Food Name	Cholesterol (mg)	Cholesterol DV	Comment
Chewing Gum	0	0%	SAFE (No Cholesterol)
Chia Seeds	0	0%	SAFE (No Cholesterol)
Chicken (Light Meat)	75	25%	High in Cholesterol
Chicken Back	87	29%	High in Cholesterol
Chickpea Flour (Besan)	0	0%	SAFE (No Cholesterol)
Chickpeas Dry	0	0%	SAFE (No Cholesterol)
Chicory Beverage	0	0%	SAFE (No Cholesterol)
Chicory Greens	0	0%	SAFE (No Cholesterol)
Chicory Roots	0	0%	SAFE (No Cholesterol)
Chili Powder	0	0%	SAFE (No Cholesterol)
Chinese Broccoli	0	0%	SAFE (No Cholesterol)
Chinese Chestnuts	0	0%	SAFE (No Cholesterol)
Chinese Pancake	0	0%	SAFE (No Cholesterol)
Chives	0	0%	SAFE (No Cholesterol)
Chocolate Almond Milk	0	0%	SAFE (No Cholesterol)
Chocolate Cake	58	19%	Medium In Cholesterol
Chocolate Dip	19	6%	Medium In Cholesterol
Chocolate Drink Powder	0	0%	SAFE (No Cholesterol)
Chorizo	63	21%	High in Cholesterol
Chuck Steak	115	38%	High in Cholesterol
Churros	7	2%	Low in Cholesterol
Chutney	0	0%	SAFE (No Cholesterol)
Cilantro	0	0%	SAFE (No Cholesterol)
Cinnamon	0	0%	SAFE (No Cholesterol)
Citrus Energy Drink	0	0%	SAFE (No Cholesterol)
Clams	30	10%	Medium In Cholesterol
Clementines	0	0%	SAFE (No Cholesterol)
Cloudberries (Alaska Native	0	0%	SAFE (No Cholesterol)
Club Soda	0	0%	SAFE (No Cholesterol)
Cocoa Butter	0	0%	SAFE (No Cholesterol)
Cocoa Dry Powder	0	0%	SAFE (No Cholesterol)
Cocoa Powder	0	0%	SAFE (No Cholesterol)
Coconut Milk	0	0%	SAFE (No Cholesterol)

Food Name	Cholesterol (mg)	Cholesterol DV	Comment
Coconut Oil	0	0%	SAFE (No Cholesterol)
Cod Liver Oil	570	190%	Very High in Cholesterol
Cod Smoked	74	25%	High in Cholesterol
Cod Steamed Or Poached	59	20%	Medium In Cholesterol
Coffee	0	0%	SAFE (No Cholesterol)
Coffee Turkish	0	0%	SAFE (No Cholesterol)
Coffeecake Cheese	85	28%	High in Cholesterol
Coleslaw (Fast Food)	4	1%	Low in Cholesterol
Coleslaw Dressing	26	9%	Medium In Cholesterol
Collards	0	0%	SAFE (No Cholesterol)
Congee	0	0%	SAFE (No Cholesterol)
Cookie Lemon Bar	68	23%	High in Cholesterol
Coriander Seed	0	0%	SAFE (No Cholesterol)
Corn Beverage	0	0%	SAFE (No Cholesterol)
Corn Cakes	0	0%	SAFE (No Cholesterol)
Corn Chips Flavored	0	0%	SAFE (No Cholesterol)
Corn Chips Flavored (Fritos)	0	0%	SAFE (No Cholesterol)
Corn Chips Plain	0	0%	SAFE (No Cholesterol)
Corn Dried	1	0%	SAFE (No Cholesterol)
Corn Dried Yellow	0	0%	SAFE (No Cholesterol)
Corn Oil	0	0%	SAFE (No Cholesterol)
Corn Pudding Home Prepare	72	24%	High in Cholesterol
Corn Relish	0	0%	SAFE (No Cholesterol)
Cornsalad	0	0%	SAFE (No Cholesterol)
Cornstarch	0	0%	SAFE (No Cholesterol)
Cottonseed Oil	0	0%	SAFE (No Cholesterol)
Couscous Dry	0	0%	SAFE (No Cholesterol)
Cowpeas (Blackeyes)	0	0%	SAFE (No Cholesterol)
Crab Cake	111	37%	High in Cholesterol
Crab Imperial	115	38%	High in Cholesterol
Crab Salad	58	19%	Medium In Cholesterol
Crabapples	0	0%	SAFE (No Cholesterol)
Cracker Meal	0	0%	SAFE (No Cholesterol)

Food Name	Cholesterol (mg)	Cholesterol DV	Comment
Crackers Milk	11	4%	Low in Cholesterol
Crackers Rice And Nuts	0	0%	SAFE (No Cholesterol)
Crackers Rusk Toast	78	26%	High in Cholesterol
Cranberries	0	0%	SAFE (No Cholesterol)
Crayfish	133	44%	High in Cholesterol
Cream Heavy	113	38%	High in Cholesterol
Cream Light	59	20%	Medium In Cholesterol
Cream Soda	0	0%	SAFE (No Cholesterol)
Cream Whipped	106	35%	High in Cholesterol
Cremini Mushrooms	0	0%	SAFE (No Cholesterol)
Crepe Chocolate Filled	62	21%	High in Cholesterol
Crepe Plain	138	46%	High in Cholesterol
Crisp Blueberry	0	0%	SAFE (No Cholesterol)
Crisp Cherry	0	0%	SAFE (No Cholesterol)
Crisp Peach	0	0%	SAFE (No Cholesterol)
Crisp Rhubarb	0	0%	SAFE (No Cholesterol)
Croissant Chocolate	54	18%	Medium In Cholesterol
Croissant Fruit	63	21%	High in Cholesterol
Crumpet	49	16%	Medium In Cholesterol
Cucumber	0	0%	SAFE (No Cholesterol)
Cumin Seed	0	0%	SAFE (No Cholesterol)
Cured Ham	62	21%	High in Cholesterol
Curry Powder	0	0%	SAFE (No Cholesterol)
Custard	72	24%	High in Cholesterol
Dandelion Greens	0	0%	SAFE (No Cholesterol)
Danish Pastry Cheese	23	8%	Medium In Cholesterol
Dasheen Boiled	0	0%	SAFE (No Cholesterol)
Date Candy	0	0%	SAFE (No Cholesterol)
Dates	0	0%	SAFE (No Cholesterol)
Decaf Coffee	0	0%	SAFE (No Cholesterol)
Dehydrated Milk	97	32%	High in Cholesterol
Dessert Dip	44	15%	Medium In Cholesterol
Dessert Pizza	9	3%	Low in Cholesterol

Food Name	Cholesterol (mg)	Cholesterol DV	Comment
Dessert Sauce	21	7%	Medium In Cholesterol
Diet Cola	0	0%	SAFE (No Cholesterol)
Diet Green Tea	0	0%	SAFE (No Cholesterol)
Dill	0	0%	SAFE (No Cholesterol)
Dip Nfs	50	17%	Medium In Cholesterol
Dock	0	0%	SAFE (No Cholesterol)
Doughnut Chocolate Cream-	25	8%	Medium In Cholesterol
Dove Fried	114	38%	High in Cholesterol
Dried Apples	0	0%	SAFE (No Cholesterol)
Dried Apricots	0	0%	SAFE (No Cholesterol)
Dried Bananas	0	0%	SAFE (No Cholesterol)
Dried Basil	0	0%	SAFE (No Cholesterol)
Dried Beechnuts	0	0%	SAFE (No Cholesterol)
Dried Blueberries (Sweetene	0	0%	SAFE (No Cholesterol)
Dried Chervil	0	0%	SAFE (No Cholesterol)
Dried Chinese Chestnuts	0	0%	SAFE (No Cholesterol)
Dried Chives	0	0%	SAFE (No Cholesterol)
Dried Coconut	0	0%	SAFE (No Cholesterol)
Dried Coconut (Unsweetene	0	0%	SAFE (No Cholesterol)
Dried Coriander	0	0%	SAFE (No Cholesterol)
Dried Cranberries (Sweetene	0	0%	SAFE (No Cholesterol)
Dried Dill Weed	0	0%	SAFE (No Cholesterol)
Dried Eggs	1630	543%	Very High in Cholesterol
Dried Figs	0	0%	SAFE (No Cholesterol)
Dried Fungi Cloud Ears	0	0%	SAFE (No Cholesterol)
Dried Ginkgo Nuts	0	0%	SAFE (No Cholesterol)
Dried Hickorynuts	0	0%	SAFE (No Cholesterol)
Dried Japanese Chestnuts	0	0%	SAFE (No Cholesterol)
Dried Jujube	0	0%	SAFE (No Cholesterol)
Dried Litchis	0	0%	SAFE (No Cholesterol)
Dried Longans	0	0%	SAFE (No Cholesterol)
Dried Lotus Seeds	0	0%	SAFE (No Cholesterol)
Dried Marjoram	0	0%	SAFE (No Cholesterol)

Food Name	Cholesterol (mg)	Cholesterol DV	Comment
Dried Oregano	0	0%	SAFE (No Cholesterol)
Dried Parsley	0	0%	SAFE (No Cholesterol)
Dried Pasilla Peppers	0	0%	SAFE (No Cholesterol)
Dried Peaches	0	0%	SAFE (No Cholesterol)
Dried Peaches (Low-Moistur	0	0%	SAFE (No Cholesterol)
Dried Pears	0	0%	SAFE (No Cholesterol)
Dried Pilinuts	0	0%	SAFE (No Cholesterol)
Dried Pine Nuts	0	0%	SAFE (No Cholesterol)
Dried Pumpkin And Squash	0	0%	SAFE (No Cholesterol)
Dried Rosemary	0	0%	SAFE (No Cholesterol)
Dried Salted Atlantic Cod	152	51%	High in Cholesterol
Dried Shiitake Mushrooms	0	0%	SAFE (No Cholesterol)
Dried Spearmint	0	0%	SAFE (No Cholesterol)
Dried Spirulina Seaweed	0	0%	SAFE (No Cholesterol)
Dried Sunflower Seeds	0	0%	SAFE (No Cholesterol)
Dried Sweet Whey Powder	6	2%	Low in Cholesterol
Dried Sweetened Mango	0	0%	SAFE (No Cholesterol)
Dried Tarragon	0	0%	SAFE (No Cholesterol)
Dried Whey Powder (Acid)	3	1%	Low in Cholesterol
Dry Roasted Almonds	0	0%	SAFE (No Cholesterol)
Dry Roasted Hazelnuts	0	0%	SAFE (No Cholesterol)
Dry Roasted Macadamia Nut	0	0%	SAFE (No Cholesterol)
Dry Roasted Peanuts	0	0%	SAFE (No Cholesterol)
Dry Roasted Pecans	0	0%	SAFE (No Cholesterol)
Dry Roasted Pistachio Nuts	0	0%	SAFE (No Cholesterol)
Dry Roasted Sunflower Seed	0	0%	SAFE (No Cholesterol)
Dry Roasted Sunflower Seed	0	0%	SAFE (No Cholesterol)
Dry-Roasted Cashews	0	0%	SAFE (No Cholesterol)
Dry-Roasted Mixed Nuts (Sa	0	0%	SAFE (No Cholesterol)
Dry-Roasted Soybeans	0	0%	SAFE (No Cholesterol)
Duck Egg	997	332%	Very High in Cholesterol
Duck Pressed Chinese	22	7%	Medium In Cholesterol
Duck Soup	41	14%	Medium In Cholesterol

Food Name	Cholesterol (mg)	Cholesterol DV	Comment
Dumpling Plain	2	1%	Low in Cholesterol
Durian	0	0%	SAFE (No Cholesterol)
Edam Cheese	89	30%	High in Cholesterol
Edamame	0	0%	SAFE (No Cholesterol)
Eel Smoked	196	65%	High in Cholesterol
Egg Bagel	24	8%	Medium In Cholesterol
Egg Creamed	169	56%	High in Cholesterol
Egg Curry	54	18%	Medium In Cholesterol
Egg Deviled	343	114%	Very High in Cholesterol
Egg Noodles	29	10%	Medium In Cholesterol
Egg Omelet	313	104%	Very High in Cholesterol
Egg Salad Sandwich	179	60%	High in Cholesterol
Egg Scrambled	426	142%	Very High in Cholesterol
Egg White Dried	0	0%	SAFE (No Cholesterol)
Egg White Powder	0	0%	SAFE (No Cholesterol)
Egg Whites	0	0%	SAFE (No Cholesterol)
Egg Yolk Dried	2307	769%	Very High in Cholesterol
Egg Yolks	1085	362%	Very High in Cholesterol
Eggnog	59	20%	Medium In Cholesterol
Eggplant	0	0%	SAFE (No Cholesterol)
Eggplant Dip	0	0%	SAFE (No Cholesterol)
Eggs	372	124%	Very High in Cholesterol
Elderberries	0	0%	SAFE (No Cholesterol)
Elk Free Range Ground Patt	70	23%	High in Cholesterol
Emu Ground	69	23%	High in Cholesterol
Emu Steak	82	27%	High in Cholesterol
Emu Top Loin Broiled	88	29%	High in Cholesterol
Endive	0	0%	SAFE (No Cholesterol)
Energy Drink	0	0%	SAFE (No Cholesterol)
English Muffins	0	0%	SAFE (No Cholesterol)
English Muffins Mixed-Grai	0	0%	SAFE (No Cholesterol)
Enoki Mushrooms	0	0%	SAFE (No Cholesterol)
Epazote	0	0%	SAFE (No Cholesterol)

Food Name	Cholesterol (mg)	Cholesterol DV	Comment
Eppaw	0	0%	SAFE (No Cholesterol)
Escarole Creamed	3	1%	Low in Cholesterol
Espresso	0	0%	SAFE (No Cholesterol)
Falafel	0	0%	SAFE (No Cholesterol)
Fat Free Cream Cheese	12	4%	Low in Cholesterol
Fat Free Ground Turkey	71	24%	High in Cholesterol
Fat Goose	100	33%	High in Cholesterol
Fat Turkey	102	34%	High in Cholesterol
Fatfree Chocolate Milk	2	1%	Low in Cholesterol
Feijoa	0	0%	SAFE (No Cholesterol)
Fennel	0	0%	SAFE (No Cholesterol)
Fennel Seed	0	0%	SAFE (No Cholesterol)
Feta Cheese	89	30%	High in Cholesterol
Fig Bars	0	0%	SAFE (No Cholesterol)
Figs	0	0%	SAFE (No Cholesterol)
Firm Tofu	0	0%	SAFE (No Cholesterol)
Fish Bluefish	59	20%	Medium In Cholesterol
Fish Broth	0	0%	SAFE (No Cholesterol)
Fish Carp	66	22%	High in Cholesterol
Fish Caviar Black And Red (	588	196%	Very High in Cholesterol
Fish Chowder	37	12%	Medium In Cholesterol
Fish Cisco	50	17%	Medium In Cholesterol
Fish Curry	9	3%	Low in Cholesterol
Fish Cusk	41	14%	Medium In Cholesterol
Fish Haddock	54	18%	Medium In Cholesterol
Fish Herring Atlantic	60	20%	Medium In Cholesterol
Fish Ling	40	13%	Medium In Cholesterol
Fish Monkfish	25	8%	Medium In Cholesterol
Fish Moochim	86	29%	High in Cholesterol
Fish Roe	374	125%	Very High in Cholesterol
Fish Roe	479	160%	Very High in Cholesterol
Fish Roughy Orange	60	20%	Medium In Cholesterol
Fish Sablefish	49	16%	Medium In Cholesterol

Food Name	Cholesterol (mg)	Cholesterol DV	Comment
Fish Salmon Chinook	50	17%	Medium In Cholesterol
Fish Salmon Chum	74	25%	High in Cholesterol
Fish Salmon Sockeye	51	17%	Medium In Cholesterol
Fish Scup	52	17%	Medium In Cholesterol
Fish Sheepshead	50	17%	Medium In Cholesterol
Fish Spot	60	20%	Medium In Cholesterol
Fish Stock	1	0%	SAFE (No Cholesterol)
Fish Surimi	30	10%	Medium In Cholesterol
Fish Swordfish	66	22%	High in Cholesterol
Fish Tilefish	50	17%	Medium In Cholesterol
Fish Timbale Or Mousse	104	35%	High in Cholesterol
Fish Tofu And Vegetables Tc	57	19%	Medium In Cholesterol
Fish Trout Brook New York	60	20%	Medium In Cholesterol
Fish Trout Mixed Species	58	19%	Medium In Cholesterol
Fish Trout Mixed Species D	74	25%	High in Cholesterol
Fish Trout Rainbow Wild	59	20%	Medium In Cholesterol
Fish Tuna Salad	13	4%	Low in Cholesterol
Flan	101	34%	High in Cholesterol
Flavored Pasta	0	0%	SAFE (No Cholesterol)
Flax Seeds	0	0%	SAFE (No Cholesterol)
Flaxseed Oil	0	0%	SAFE (No Cholesterol)
Florida Avocados	0	0%	SAFE (No Cholesterol)
Florida Grapefruit	0	0%	SAFE (No Cholesterol)
Florida Oranges	0	0%	SAFE (No Cholesterol)
Flounder Smoked	109	36%	High in Cholesterol
Fontina Cheese	116	39%	High in Cholesterol
Fortified Silken Tofu	0	0%	SAFE (No Cholesterol)
Forunte Cookies	2	1%	Low in Cholesterol
Frankfurter Beef Heated	58	19%	Medium In Cholesterol
Frankfurter Low Sodium	61	20%	High in Cholesterol
Frankfurter Meat	77	26%	High in Cholesterol
French Bread	0	0%	SAFE (No Cholesterol)
French Fries	0	0%	SAFE (No Cholesterol)

Food Name	Cholesterol (mg)	Cholesterol DV	Comment
French Toast Nfs	160	53%	High in Cholesterol
French Toast Plain	160	53%	High in Cholesterol
Fresh Water Bass	68	23%	High in Cholesterol
Fried Bread Puerto Rican Sty	56	19%	Medium In Cholesterol
Fried Calamari	260	87%	High in Cholesterol
Fried Eggs	401	134%	Very High in Cholesterol
Fritter Apple	79	26%	High in Cholesterol
Fritter Banana	54	18%	Medium In Cholesterol
Fritter Berry	65	22%	High in Cholesterol
Frog Legs	50	17%	Medium In Cholesterol
Frog Legs Ns As To Cooking	81	27%	High in Cholesterol
Frog Legs Steamed	63	21%	High in Cholesterol
Frozen Coffee Drink	4	1%	Low in Cholesterol
Frozen Coffee Drink Decaffe	4	1%	Low in Cholesterol
Frozen Daiquiri	0	0%	SAFE (No Cholesterol)
Frozen Raspberries	0	0%	SAFE (No Cholesterol)
Frozen Stberries	0	0%	SAFE (No Cholesterol)
Gala Apples	0	0%	SAFE (No Cholesterol)
Garden Cress	0	0%	SAFE (No Cholesterol)
Garlic	0	0%	SAFE (No Cholesterol)
Garlic Powder	0	0%	SAFE (No Cholesterol)
Garlic Sauce	19	6%	Medium In Cholesterol
Gelatin Dessert	0	0%	SAFE (No Cholesterol)
Gelatin Dessert With Fruit	0	0%	SAFE (No Cholesterol)
Gelatin Snacks	0	0%	SAFE (No Cholesterol)
Gluten Free Corn Noodles	0	0%	SAFE (No Cholesterol)
Gnocchi Cheese	63	21%	High in Cholesterol
Gnocchi Potato	16	5%	Medium In Cholesterol
Goat	57	19%	Medium In Cholesterol
Goat Baked	74	25%	High in Cholesterol
Goat Boiled	74	25%	High in Cholesterol
Goat Fried	73	24%	High in Cholesterol
Goat Milk	11	4%	Low in Cholesterol

Food Name	Cholesterol (mg)	Cholesterol DV	Comment
Golden Cadillac	44	15%	Medium In Cholesterol
Gooseberries	0	0%	SAFE (No Cholesterol)
Goulash Nfs	54	18%	Medium In Cholesterol
Grape Juice	0	0%	SAFE (No Cholesterol)
Grape Leaves	0	0%	SAFE (No Cholesterol)
Grape Soda	0	0%	SAFE (No Cholesterol)
Grapefruit	0	0%	SAFE (No Cholesterol)
Grapefruit Juice	0	0%	SAFE (No Cholesterol)
Grapes	0	0%	SAFE (No Cholesterol)
Grapes Canned	0	0%	SAFE (No Cholesterol)
Grapeseed Oil	0	0%	SAFE (No Cholesterol)
Grated Parmesan	86	29%	High in Cholesterol
Gravy Giblet	51	17%	Medium In Cholesterol
Gravy Redeye	5	2%	Low in Cholesterol
Greek Yogurt (Plain)	13	4%	Low in Cholesterol
Green Bell Peppers	0	0%	SAFE (No Cholesterol)
Green Cauliflower	0	0%	SAFE (No Cholesterol)
Green Chili Peppers	0	0%	SAFE (No Cholesterol)
Green Leaf Lettuce	0	0%	SAFE (No Cholesterol)
Green Olives	0	0%	SAFE (No Cholesterol)
Green Snap Beans	0	0%	SAFE (No Cholesterol)
Green Soybeans	0	0%	SAFE (No Cholesterol)
Green Tea	0	0%	SAFE (No Cholesterol)
Green Tomatoes	0	0%	SAFE (No Cholesterol)
Ground Allspice	0	0%	SAFE (No Cholesterol)
Ground Beef	71	24%	High in Cholesterol
Ground Cloves	0	0%	SAFE (No Cholesterol)
Ground Ginger	0	0%	SAFE (No Cholesterol)
Ground Mace	0	0%	SAFE (No Cholesterol)
Ground Meat Nfs	87	29%	High in Cholesterol
Ground Mustard Seed	0	0%	SAFE (No Cholesterol)
Ground Nutmeg	0	0%	SAFE (No Cholesterol)
Ground Sage	0	0%	SAFE (No Cholesterol)

Food Name	Cholesterol (mg)	Cholesterol DV	Comment
Ground Savory	0	0%	SAFE (No Cholesterol)
Ground Turmeric	0	0%	SAFE (No Cholesterol)
Groundcherries	0	0%	SAFE (No Cholesterol)
Gruyere Cheese	110	37%	High in Cholesterol
Guava Paste	0	0%	SAFE (No Cholesterol)
Guavas	0	0%	SAFE (No Cholesterol)
Halavah Plain	0	0%	SAFE (No Cholesterol)
Halibut Smoked	118	39%	High in Cholesterol
Halvah Plain	0	0%	SAFE (No Cholesterol)
Ham Minced	70	23%	High in Cholesterol
Hamburger Nfs	37	12%	Medium In Cholesterol
Haupia	0	0%	SAFE (No Cholesterol)
Hazelnut Oil	0	0%	SAFE (No Cholesterol)
Hazelnuts	0	0%	SAFE (No Cholesterol)
Herring Oil	766	255%	Very High in Cholesterol
Herring Pickled In Cream Sa	22	7%	Medium In Cholesterol
Hoisin Sauce	3	1%	Low in Cholesterol
Honey	0	0%	SAFE (No Cholesterol)
Honey Butter	86	29%	High in Cholesterol
Horseradish	0	0%	SAFE (No Cholesterol)
Hot Cocoa	8	3%	Low in Cholesterol
Hot Dog Relish	0	0%	SAFE (No Cholesterol)
Hot Sauce	0	0%	SAFE (No Cholesterol)
Hummus Flavored	0	0%	SAFE (No Cholesterol)
Hummus Plain	0	0%	SAFE (No Cholesterol)
Hungarian Peppers	0	0%	SAFE (No Cholesterol)
Hush Puppies	0	0%	SAFE (No Cholesterol)
Ice Cream Bar Cake Covered	58	19%	Medium In Cholesterol
Ice Cream Fried	34	11%	Medium In Cholesterol
Ice Creams Vanilla Fat Free	0	0%	SAFE (No Cholesterol)
Instant Soup Noodle	5	2%	Low in Cholesterol
Irish Coffee	7	2%	Low in Cholesterol
Jackfruit	0	0%	SAFE (No Cholesterol)

Food Name	Cholesterol (mg)	Cholesterol DV	Comment
Jellies	0	0%	SAFE (No Cholesterol)
Jellybeans	0	0%	SAFE (No Cholesterol)
Jews Ear	0	0%	SAFE (No Cholesterol)
Kale	0	0%	SAFE (No Cholesterol)
Kamut	0	0%	SAFE (No Cholesterol)
Kanpyo	0	0%	SAFE (No Cholesterol)
Ketchup	0	0%	SAFE (No Cholesterol)
Kidney	710	237%	Very High in Cholesterol
Kidney Bean Sprouts	0	0%	SAFE (No Cholesterol)
Kidney Beans	0	0%	SAFE (No Cholesterol)
Kimchi	0	0%	SAFE (No Cholesterol)
Kiwifruit	0	0%	SAFE (No Cholesterol)
Knish Cheese	83	28%	High in Cholesterol
Knish Meat	95	32%	High in Cholesterol
Knish Potato	85	28%	High in Cholesterol
Kohlrabi	0	0%	SAFE (No Cholesterol)
Lamb Liver	493	164%	Very High in Cholesterol
Lamb Ribs	97	32%	High in Cholesterol
Lamb Sirloin	92	31%	High in Cholesterol
Lambsquarters	0	0%	SAFE (No Cholesterol)
Lard	95	32%	High in Cholesterol
Leeks	0	0%	SAFE (No Cholesterol)
Lemon Juice	0	0%	SAFE (No Cholesterol)
Lemon Peel	0	0%	SAFE (No Cholesterol)
Lemon Pie Filling	115	38%	High in Cholesterol
Lemons	0	0%	SAFE (No Cholesterol)
Lentil Sprouts	0	0%	SAFE (No Cholesterol)
Lentils	0	0%	SAFE (No Cholesterol)
Lima Beans	0	0%	SAFE (No Cholesterol)
Limburger Cheese	90	30%	High in Cholesterol
Lime Juice	0	0%	SAFE (No Cholesterol)
Lime Souffle	226	75%	High in Cholesterol
Limes	0	0%	SAFE (No Cholesterol)

Food Name	Cholesterol (mg)	Cholesterol DV	Comment
Litchis	0	0%	SAFE (No Cholesterol)
Liver Dumpling	335	112%	Very High in Cholesterol
Loaf Lentil	0	0%	SAFE (No Cholesterol)
Lobster	146	49%	High in Cholesterol
Lobster Salad	85	28%	High in Cholesterol
Lobster Sauce	69	23%	High in Cholesterol
Longans	0	0%	SAFE (No Cholesterol)
Loquats	0	0%	SAFE (No Cholesterol)
Lotus Root	0	0%	SAFE (No Cholesterol)
Lotus Seeds	0	0%	SAFE (No Cholesterol)
Low Calorie Cola	0	0%	SAFE (No Cholesterol)
Low-Fat Milk 1%	5	2%	Low in Cholesterol
Low-Fat Milk 2%	8	3%	Low in Cholesterol
Low-Fat Yogurt	6	2%	Low in Cholesterol
Lowfat Buttermilk	4	1%	Low in Cholesterol
Lupin Beans	0	0%	SAFE (No Cholesterol)
Macadamia Nuts	0	0%	SAFE (No Cholesterol)
Mackerel	62	21%	High in Cholesterol
Mackerel Pickled	40	13%	Medium In Cholesterol
Mackerel Smoked	60	20%	Medium In Cholesterol
Mangos	0	0%	SAFE (No Cholesterol)
Manhattan Clam Chowder	6	2%	Low in Cholesterol
Margarine	0	0%	SAFE (No Cholesterol)
Margarine (Unsalted)	0	0%	SAFE (No Cholesterol)
Margarita	0	0%	SAFE (No Cholesterol)
Melon Balls	0	0%	SAFE (No Cholesterol)
Melon Banana (Navajo)	0	0%	SAFE (No Cholesterol)
Menhaden Oil	521	174%	Very High in Cholesterol
Menudo Soup	27	9%	Medium In Cholesterol
Menudo Soup Home Recipe	32	11%	Medium In Cholesterol
Meringues	0	0%	SAFE (No Cholesterol)
Millet	0	0%	SAFE (No Cholesterol)
Millet Flour	0	0%	SAFE (No Cholesterol)

Food Name	Cholesterol (mg)	Cholesterol DV	Comment
Minestrone	1	0%	SAFE (No Cholesterol)
Miso	0	0%	SAFE (No Cholesterol)
Miso Sauce	0	0%	SAFE (No Cholesterol)
Mixed Seeds	0	0%	SAFE (No Cholesterol)
Mojito	0	0%	SAFE (No Cholesterol)
Molasses	0	0%	SAFE (No Cholesterol)
Molasses Cookies	0	0%	SAFE (No Cholesterol)
Monterey Cheese	89	30%	High in Cholesterol
Moo Goo Gai Pan	17	6%	Medium In Cholesterol
Mozzarella	79	26%	High in Cholesterol
Muffin Carrot	39	13%	Medium In Cholesterol
Muffin Cheese	69	23%	High in Cholesterol
Muffin Chocolate	46	15%	Medium In Cholesterol
Muffin Plain	48	16%	Medium In Cholesterol
Muffin Pumpkin	38	13%	Medium In Cholesterol
Muffin Wheat	53	18%	Medium In Cholesterol
Mulberries	0	0%	SAFE (No Cholesterol)
Mushrooms Pickled	0	0%	SAFE (No Cholesterol)
Mustard Greens	0	0%	SAFE (No Cholesterol)
Mustard Oil	0	0%	SAFE (No Cholesterol)
Mustard Spinach	0	0%	SAFE (No Cholesterol)
Navel Oranges	0	0%	SAFE (No Cholesterol)
Navy Beans	0	0%	SAFE (No Cholesterol)
Nectarines	0	0%	SAFE (No Cholesterol)
Non-Fat Yogurt	2	1%	Low in Cholesterol
Noodles	29	10%	Medium In Cholesterol
Noodles Egg Enriched With	29	10%	Medium In Cholesterol
Nopales	0	0%	SAFE (No Cholesterol)
Nougat Chocolate Covered	6	2%	Low in Cholesterol
Nougat With Almonds	0	0%	SAFE (No Cholesterol)
Nuts Acorns	0	0%	SAFE (No Cholesterol)
Nuts Almond Butter Plain W	0	0%	SAFE (No Cholesterol)
Oat Bran	0	0%	SAFE (No Cholesterol)

Food Name	Cholesterol (mg)	Cholesterol DV	Comment
Oatmeal Cookies	0	0%	SAFE (No Cholesterol)
Octopus	96	32%	High in Cholesterol
Octopus Dried	182	61%	High in Cholesterol
Octopus Dried Boiled	96	32%	High in Cholesterol
Oheloberries	0	0%	SAFE (No Cholesterol)
Oil Babassu	0	0%	SAFE (No Cholesterol)
Oil Nutmeg Butter	0	0%	SAFE (No Cholesterol)
Oil Oat	0	0%	SAFE (No Cholesterol)
Oil Sheanut	0	0%	SAFE (No Cholesterol)
Okara	0	0%	SAFE (No Cholesterol)
Olive Oil	0	0%	SAFE (No Cholesterol)
Olives	0	0%	SAFE (No Cholesterol)
Onion Powder	0	0%	SAFE (No Cholesterol)
Onions	0	0%	SAFE (No Cholesterol)
Orange Juice	0	0%	SAFE (No Cholesterol)
Orange Soda	0	0%	SAFE (No Cholesterol)
Oranges	0	0%	SAFE (No Cholesterol)
Oriental Radishes	0	0%	SAFE (No Cholesterol)
Ostrich	82	27%	High in Cholesterol
Ostrich Steak	97	32%	High in Cholesterol
Osyter Sauce	0	0%	SAFE (No Cholesterol)
Palm Oil	0	0%	SAFE (No Cholesterol)
Pancakes Plain	60	20%	Medium In Cholesterol
Pancakes Pumpkin	50	17%	Medium In Cholesterol
Pannetone	59	20%	Medium In Cholesterol
Papad	4	1%	Low in Cholesterol
Papaya	0	0%	SAFE (No Cholesterol)
Paprika	0	0%	SAFE (No Cholesterol)
Parsley	0	0%	SAFE (No Cholesterol)
Parsnips	0	0%	SAFE (No Cholesterol)
Pasta	0	0%	SAFE (No Cholesterol)
Pasta Sauce	2	1%	Low in Cholesterol
Pastrami Turkey	68	23%	High in Cholesterol

Food Name	Cholesterol (mg)	Cholesterol DV	Comment
Pea Salad	8	3%	Low in Cholesterol
Pea Sprouts	0	0%	SAFE (No Cholesterol)
Peach Nectar	0	0%	SAFE (No Cholesterol)
Peanut Bar	0	0%	SAFE (No Cholesterol)
Peanut Flour Low Fat	0	0%	SAFE (No Cholesterol)
Peanut Oil	0	0%	SAFE (No Cholesterol)
Pears	0	0%	SAFE (No Cholesterol)
Peas	0	0%	SAFE (No Cholesterol)
Pecans	0	0%	SAFE (No Cholesterol)
Peppermint	0	0%	SAFE (No Cholesterol)
Pepperoni	97	32%	High in Cholesterol
Pepperpot Soup	20	7%	Medium In Cholesterol
Pesto	0	0%	SAFE (No Cholesterol)
Pesto Sauce	16	5%	Medium In Cholesterol
Pickled Sausage	70	23%	High in Cholesterol
Pie Oatmeal	67	22%	High in Cholesterol
Pie Peach	0	0%	SAFE (No Cholesterol)
Pie Squash	38	13%	Medium In Cholesterol
Pimiento	0	0%	SAFE (No Cholesterol)
Pineapple	0	0%	SAFE (No Cholesterol)
Pineapple Dried	0	0%	SAFE (No Cholesterol)
Pistachio Nuts	0	0%	SAFE (No Cholesterol)
Pita Bread	0	0%	SAFE (No Cholesterol)
Pitanga	0	0%	SAFE (No Cholesterol)
Plain Yogurt	13	4%	Low in Cholesterol
Plums	0	0%	SAFE (No Cholesterol)
Pomegranates	0	0%	SAFE (No Cholesterol)
Popcorn	0	0%	SAFE (No Cholesterol)
Popeyes Coleslaw	7	2%	Low in Cholesterol
Poppy Seeds	0	0%	SAFE (No Cholesterol)
Poppyseed Oil	0	0%	SAFE (No Cholesterol)
Potato Baked	0	0%	SAFE (No Cholesterol)
Potato Baked Peel Eaten	0	0%	SAFE (No Cholesterol)

Food Name	Cholesterol (mg)	Cholesterol DV	Comment
Potato Chowder	12	4%	Low in Cholesterol
Potato Flour	0	0%	SAFE (No Cholesterol)
Potato Pudding	58	19%	Medium In Cholesterol
Pretzels Soft Nfs	3	1%	Low in Cholesterol
Protein Powder Soy Based	0	0%	SAFE (No Cholesterol)
Protein Powder Whey Based	16	5%	Medium In Cholesterol
Prune Dried With Sugar	0	0%	SAFE (No Cholesterol)
Prune Puree	0	0%	SAFE (No Cholesterol)
Prune Whip	0	0%	SAFE (No Cholesterol)
Prunes (Dried Plums)	0	0%	SAFE (No Cholesterol)
Pudding Bread	55	18%	Medium In Cholesterol
Pummelo	0	0%	SAFE (No Cholesterol)
Pumpkin	0	0%	SAFE (No Cholesterol)
Pumpkin Flowers	0	0%	SAFE (No Cholesterol)
Pumpkin Seeds Salted	0	0%	SAFE (No Cholesterol)
Purslane	0	0%	SAFE (No Cholesterol)
Quail	86	29%	High in Cholesterol
Queen Crab	55	18%	Medium In Cholesterol
Quesadilla Just Cheese From	37	12%	Medium In Cholesterol
Queso Fresco	69	23%	High in Cholesterol
Quinoa	0	0%	SAFE (No Cholesterol)
Radicchio	0	0%	SAFE (No Cholesterol)
Radish Sprouts	0	0%	SAFE (No Cholesterol)
Radishes	0	0%	SAFE (No Cholesterol)
Radishes Hawaiian Style Pic	0	0%	SAFE (No Cholesterol)
Rainbow Trout	59	20%	Medium In Cholesterol
Raisins	0	0%	SAFE (No Cholesterol)
Raspberries	0	0%	SAFE (No Cholesterol)
Ratatouille	0	0%	SAFE (No Cholesterol)
Recaito	0	0%	SAFE (No Cholesterol)
Red Bell Peppers	0	0%	SAFE (No Cholesterol)
Red Cabbage	0	0%	SAFE (No Cholesterol)
Red Chili Peppers	0	0%	SAFE (No Cholesterol)

Food Name	Cholesterol (mg)	Cholesterol DV	Comment
Red Leaf Lettuce	0	0%	SAFE (No Cholesterol)
Reeses Bites	7	2%	Low in Cholesterol
Rhubarb	0	0%	SAFE (No Cholesterol)
Rice Bran	0	0%	SAFE (No Cholesterol)
Rice Bran Oil	0	0%	SAFE (No Cholesterol)
Rice Crackers	0	0%	SAFE (No Cholesterol)
Rice Croquette	39	13%	Medium In Cholesterol
Rice Dressing	0	0%	SAFE (No Cholesterol)
Rice Paper	0	0%	SAFE (No Cholesterol)
Ricotta Cheese	49	16%	Medium In Cholesterol
Roast Duck	89	30%	High in Cholesterol
Roasted Ham	94	31%	High in Cholesterol
Roll Garlic	4	1%	Low in Cholesterol
Rosemary	0	0%	SAFE (No Cholesterol)
Rowal	0	0%	SAFE (No Cholesterol)
Rye Bread	0	0%	SAFE (No Cholesterol)
Safflower Seeds	0	0%	SAFE (No Cholesterol)
Saffron	0	0%	SAFE (No Cholesterol)
Salami	80	27%	High in Cholesterol
Salmon Cake Or Patty	69	23%	High in Cholesterol
Salmon Canned	59	20%	Medium In Cholesterol
Salmon Dried	144	48%	High in Cholesterol
Salmon Loaf	103	34%	High in Cholesterol
Salmon Oil	485	162%	Very High in Cholesterol
Salted Butter	215	72%	High in Cholesterol
Sardine Oil	710	237%	Very High in Cholesterol
Sardines Dried	154	51%	High in Cholesterol
Sausage Gravy	25	8%	Medium In Cholesterol
Savoy Cabbage	0	0%	SAFE (No Cholesterol)
Scallop Squash	0	0%	SAFE (No Cholesterol)
Scallops	41	14%	Medium In Cholesterol
Scone	102	34%	High in Cholesterol
Seafood Salad	92	31%	High in Cholesterol

Food Name	Cholesterol (mg)	Cholesterol DV	Comment
Seafood Souffle	148	49%	High in Cholesterol
Seaweed	0	0%	SAFE (No Cholesterol)
Seaweed Soup	6	2%	Low in Cholesterol
Sesame Butter (Tahini)	0	0%	SAFE (No Cholesterol)
Sesame Crunch	0	0%	SAFE (No Cholesterol)
Sesame Oil	0	0%	SAFE (No Cholesterol)
Sesame Seed Dressing	0	0%	SAFE (No Cholesterol)
Sesame Seeds	0	0%	SAFE (No Cholesterol)
Shallots	0	0%	SAFE (No Cholesterol)
Shav Soup	65	22%	High in Cholesterol
Shortening	56	19%	Medium In Cholesterol
Shredded Parmesan	72	24%	High in Cholesterol
Shrimp Curry	33	11%	Medium In Cholesterol
Shrimp Dried	638	213%	Very High in Cholesterol
Shrimp Salad	133	44%	High in Cholesterol
Silk (Soy Milk)	0	0%	SAFE (No Cholesterol)
Skim Milk	2	1%	Low in Cholesterol
Smoked Salmon	23	8%	Medium In Cholesterol
Smoked Sturgeon	80	27%	High in Cholesterol
Smoked Whitefish	33	11%	Medium In Cholesterol
Snow Peas	0	0%	SAFE (No Cholesterol)
Snowpea	0	0%	SAFE (No Cholesterol)
Soft Goat Cheese	46	15%	Medium In Cholesterol
Soft Pretzels	0	0%	SAFE (No Cholesterol)
Soft Tofu	0	0%	SAFE (No Cholesterol)
Soup Fruit	0	0%	SAFE (No Cholesterol)
Soursop	0	0%	SAFE (No Cholesterol)
Soy Milk	0	0%	SAFE (No Cholesterol)
Soy Sauce	0	0%	SAFE (No Cholesterol)
Soybean Lecithin	0	0%	SAFE (No Cholesterol)
Soybean Oil	0	0%	SAFE (No Cholesterol)
Soybean Sprouts	0	0%	SAFE (No Cholesterol)
Soychips	0	0%	SAFE (No Cholesterol)

Food Name	Cholesterol (mg)	Cholesterol DV	Comment
Spaghetti Squash	0	0%	SAFE (No Cholesterol)
Spanish Stew	15	5%	Low in Cholesterol
Spinach	0	0%	SAFE (No Cholesterol)
Spinach Soup	2	1%	Low in Cholesterol
Spirulina	0	0%	SAFE (No Cholesterol)
Split Peas	0	0%	SAFE (No Cholesterol)
Spoonbread	78	26%	High in Cholesterol
Spring Onions	0	0%	SAFE (No Cholesterol)
Squash Summer Souffle	92	31%	High in Cholesterol
Squash Zucchini Baby	0	0%	SAFE (No Cholesterol)
Squid	233	78%	High in Cholesterol
Squirrel	120	40%	High in Cholesterol
Sriracha	0	0%	SAFE (No Cholesterol)
Strudel Cheese	62	21%	High in Cholesterol
Strudel Cherry	12	4%	Low in Cholesterol
Strudel Peach	13	4%	Low in Cholesterol
Strudel Pineapple	14	5%	Low in Cholesterol
Sturgeon Steamed	75	25%	High in Cholesterol
Subway Tuna Sub	28	9%	Medium In Cholesterol
Succotash	0	0%	SAFE (No Cholesterol)
Sugar	0	0%	SAFE (No Cholesterol)
Sugar Apples	0	0%	SAFE (No Cholesterol)
Sugars Maple	0	0%	SAFE (No Cholesterol)
Sugars Powdered	0	0%	SAFE (No Cholesterol)
Summer Squash	0	0%	SAFE (No Cholesterol)
Sushi	4	1%	Low in Cholesterol
Swamp Cabbage	0	0%	SAFE (No Cholesterol)
Sweet Chocolate	0	0%	SAFE (No Cholesterol)
Sweet Potatoes	0	0%	SAFE (No Cholesterol)
Sweet Yellow Peppers	0	0%	SAFE (No Cholesterol)
Swiss Chard	0	0%	SAFE (No Cholesterol)
Swiss Cheese	93	31%	High in Cholesterol
Swiss Steak	31	10%	Medium In Cholesterol

Food Name	Cholesterol (mg)	Cholesterol DV	Comment
Syrup Cane	0	0%	SAFE (No Cholesterol)
Syrup Dietetic	0	0%	SAFE (No Cholesterol)
Syrups Maple	0	0%	SAFE (No Cholesterol)
Syrups Sorghum	0	0%	SAFE (No Cholesterol)
Tabasco Sauce	0	0%	SAFE (No Cholesterol)
Tabbouleh	0	0%	SAFE (No Cholesterol)
Table Salt	0	0%	SAFE (No Cholesterol)
Taco Shell Flour	0	0%	SAFE (No Cholesterol)
Taffy	0	0%	SAFE (No Cholesterol)
Tamari	0	0%	SAFE (No Cholesterol)
Tamarinds	0	0%	SAFE (No Cholesterol)
Tangerine Juice	0	0%	SAFE (No Cholesterol)
Tangerines	0	0%	SAFE (No Cholesterol)
Tap Water	0	0%	SAFE (No Cholesterol)
Taro	0	0%	SAFE (No Cholesterol)
Tea Green Brewed Decaffein	0	0%	SAFE (No Cholesterol)
Tea Green Brewed Regular	0	0%	SAFE (No Cholesterol)
Tea Hot Chai With Milk	4	1%	Low in Cholesterol
Tea Instant Lemon Diet	0	0%	SAFE (No Cholesterol)
Thyme (Fresh)	0	0%	SAFE (No Cholesterol)
Tilsit Cheese	102	34%	High in Cholesterol
Tiramisu	123	41%	High in Cholesterol
Toasted Bagels	0	0%	SAFE (No Cholesterol)
Toffee Plain	7	2%	Low in Cholesterol
Tofu Yogurt	0	0%	SAFE (No Cholesterol)
Tomatillos	0	0%	SAFE (No Cholesterol)
Tomato Aspic	0	0%	SAFE (No Cholesterol)
Tomato Powder	0	0%	SAFE (No Cholesterol)
Tomato Relish	0	0%	SAFE (No Cholesterol)
Tomatoes	0	0%	SAFE (No Cholesterol)
Tomatoseed Oil	0	0%	SAFE (No Cholesterol)
Tonic Water	0	0%	SAFE (No Cholesterol)
Toppings Pineapple	0	0%	SAFE (No Cholesterol)

Food Name	Cholesterol (mg)	Cholesterol DV	Comment
Toppings Stberry	0	0%	SAFE (No Cholesterol)
Trail Mix	4	1%	Low in Cholesterol
Tripe	127	42%	High in Cholesterol
Triticale	0	0%	SAFE (No Cholesterol)
Truffles	41	14%	Medium In Cholesterol
Tuna Fresh Dried	122	41%	High in Cholesterol
Tuna Fresh Smoked	60	20%	Medium In Cholesterol
Tuna Loaf	83	28%	High in Cholesterol
Tuna Pot Pie	12	4%	Low in Cholesterol
Turkey Back	86	29%	High in Cholesterol
Turkey Ground	92	31%	High in Cholesterol
Turkey Hotdog	77	26%	High in Cholesterol
Turkey Nuggets	60	20%	Medium In Cholesterol
Turnip Greens	0	0%	SAFE (No Cholesterol)
Turnip Pickled	0	0%	SAFE (No Cholesterol)
Turnips	0	0%	SAFE (No Cholesterol)
Turnover Guava	0	0%	SAFE (No Cholesterol)
Un Oats	0	0%	SAFE (No Cholesterol)
Un Whole-Grain Cornmeal	0	0%	SAFE (No Cholesterol)
Unsalted Butter	215	72%	High in Cholesterol
Unsweetened Rice Milk	0	0%	SAFE (No Cholesterol)
Unsweetened Soy Milk	0	0%	SAFE (No Cholesterol)
Vanilla Extract	0	0%	SAFE (No Cholesterol)
Vanilla Soy Milk	0	0%	SAFE (No Cholesterol)
Veal Bratwurst	79	26%	High in Cholesterol
Veal Breaded With Spaghett	23	8%	Medium In Cholesterol
Veal Cordon Bleu	95	32%	High in Cholesterol
Veal Ground	49	16%	Medium In Cholesterol
Veal Leg Top Roast	135	45%	High in Cholesterol
Veal Marsala	68	23%	High in Cholesterol
Veal Parmigiana	66	22%	High in Cholesterol
Veal Scallopini	67	22%	High in Cholesterol
Vegetable Broth	0	0%	SAFE (No Cholesterol)

Food Name	Cholesterol (mg)	Cholesterol DV	Comment
Vegetable Chips	0	0%	SAFE (No Cholesterol)
Vegetable Curry	0	0%	SAFE (No Cholesterol)
Vegetable Relish	0	0%	SAFE (No Cholesterol)
Vegetable Shortening	0	0%	SAFE (No Cholesterol)
Vegetable Soup	0	0%	SAFE (No Cholesterol)
Vegetable Tempura	38	13%	Medium In Cholesterol
Vegetarian Fillets	0	0%	SAFE (No Cholesterol)
Vegetarian Stew	5	2%	Low in Cholesterol
Vinespinach	0	0%	SAFE (No Cholesterol)
Vital Wheat Gluten	0	0%	SAFE (No Cholesterol)
Vitamin Fortified Water	0	0%	SAFE (No Cholesterol)
Waffle Buttermilk Frozen Re	16	5%	Medium In Cholesterol
Waffle Buttermilk Frozen Re	13	4%	Low in Cholesterol
Waffle Chocolate	64	21%	High in Cholesterol
Waffle Chocolate From Fast	61	20%	High in Cholesterol
Waffle Chocolate From Froz	14	5%	Low in Cholesterol
Waffle Cinnamon	70	23%	High in Cholesterol
Waffle Cornmeal	52	17%	Medium In Cholesterol
Waffle Fruit	55	18%	Medium In Cholesterol
Waffle Plain	70	23%	High in Cholesterol
Waffles Gluten-Free Frozen I	0	0%	SAFE (No Cholesterol)
Wakame	0	0%	SAFE (No Cholesterol)
Walnut Oil	0	0%	SAFE (No Cholesterol)
Walnuts	0	0%	SAFE (No Cholesterol)
Walnuts Honey Roasted	0	0%	SAFE (No Cholesterol)
Wasabi	0	0%	SAFE (No Cholesterol)
Wasabi Root	0	0%	SAFE (No Cholesterol)
Water Chestnut	0	0%	SAFE (No Cholesterol)
Water Non-Carbonated	0	0%	SAFE (No Cholesterol)
Watercress	0	0%	SAFE (No Cholesterol)
Watercress Broth With Shrin	39	13%	Medium In Cholesterol
Watermelon	0	0%	SAFE (No Cholesterol)
Well Water	0	0%	SAFE (No Cholesterol)

Food Name	Cholesterol (mg)	Cholesterol DV	Comment
Welsh Rarebit	25	8%	Medium In Cholesterol
Wheat Bread	0	0%	SAFE (No Cholesterol)
Wheat Durum	0	0%	SAFE (No Cholesterol)
Wheat Germ Crude	0	0%	SAFE (No Cholesterol)
Wheat Germ Oil	0	0%	SAFE (No Cholesterol)
Wheat Sprouted	0	0%	SAFE (No Cholesterol)
Wheatena Dry	0	0%	SAFE (No Cholesterol)
Whelk	130	43%	High in Cholesterol
Whey Acid Fluid	1	0%	SAFE (No Cholesterol)
Whey Protein Powder Isolate	12	4%	Low in Cholesterol
Whipped Butter (Salted)	225	75%	High in Cholesterol
Whipped Cream	76	25%	High in Cholesterol
Whiskey	0	0%	SAFE (No Cholesterol)
White Bread	0	0%	SAFE (No Cholesterol)
White Chocolate	21	7%	Medium In Cholesterol
White Grapefruit	0	0%	SAFE (No Cholesterol)
White Grapefruit Juice	0	0%	SAFE (No Cholesterol)
White Pepper	0	0%	SAFE (No Cholesterol)
White Rice	0	0%	SAFE (No Cholesterol)
Whitefish	60	20%	Medium In Cholesterol
Whole Milk	10	3%	Low in Cholesterol
Whole Wheat Bread	0	0%	SAFE (No Cholesterol)
Whole Wheat Pasta	0	0%	SAFE (No Cholesterol)
Whole Wheat Pita	0	0%	SAFE (No Cholesterol)
Wild Rice	0	0%	SAFE (No Cholesterol)
Winter Squash	0	0%	SAFE (No Cholesterol)
Witloof Chicory	0	0%	SAFE (No Cholesterol)
Worcestershire Sauce	0	0%	SAFE (No Cholesterol)
Yam	0	0%	SAFE (No Cholesterol)
Yambean (Jicama)	0	0%	SAFE (No Cholesterol)
Yardlong Bean Boiled Drain	0	0%	SAFE (No Cholesterol)
Yautia	0	0%	SAFE (No Cholesterol)
Yeast Extract Spread	0	0%	SAFE (No Cholesterol)

Food Name	Cholesterol (mg)	Cholesterol DV	Comment
Yellow Mustard	0	0%	SAFE (No Cholesterol)
Yellow Onions	0	0%	SAFE (No Cholesterol)
Yellow Peaches	0	0%	SAFE (No Cholesterol)
Yellow Snap Beans	0	0%	SAFE (No Cholesterol)
Yellow Sweet Corn	0	0%	SAFE (No Cholesterol)
Yellow Tomatoes	0	0%	SAFE (No Cholesterol)
Yellowfin Tuna	39	13%	Medium In Cholesterol
Yellowtail	55	18%	Medium In Cholesterol
Yogurt Coconut Milk	0	0%	SAFE (No Cholesterol)
Yogurt Dressing	58	19%	Medium In Cholesterol
Yogurt Liquid	4	1%	Low in Cholesterol
Yokan	0	0%	SAFE (No Cholesterol)
York Bites	1	0%	SAFE (No Cholesterol)
Yuca Fries	0	0%	SAFE (No Cholesterol)
Zabaglione	313	104%	Very High in Cholesterol
Zante Currants	0	0%	SAFE (No Cholesterol)
Zucchini	0	0%	SAFE (No Cholesterol)
Zucchini Pickled	0	0%	SAFE (No Cholesterol)
Zucchini Soup Cream Of Pre	3	1%	Low in Cholesterol
Zwieback	8	3%	Low in Cholesterol

The Safe grocery list of low cholesterol foods

Table of Contents

The Safe grocery list of low cholesterol foods......................1

    Vegetables 3

    Baked Foods... 4

    Beverages 5

    Dairy and Egg Products.. 6

    Fats and Oils 7

    Sweets.. 8

    Soups and Sauces 10

    Spices and Herbs 11

    Snacks 12

    Nuts and Seeds 13

    Grains and Pasta 14

    FRUITS 15

    Lentils and Beans 18

    18

Vegetables

- Artichokes
- Beet Greens
- Beets
- Broccoli Raab
- Burdock Root
- Butternut Squash
- Cabbage
- Carrots
- Cauliflower
- Celeriac
- Celery
- Chayote
- Chinese Broccoli
- Chrysanthemum
- Collards
- Crookneck Summer Squash
- Dandelion Greens
- Eggplant
- Escarole
- Green Cauliflower
- Green Peas
- Kale
- Leeks
- Lentil Sprouts
- Lima Beans
- Lotus Root
- Malabar Spinach
- Mustard Greens
- Okra
- Onions
- Parsnips
- Pumpkin
- Pumpkin Flowers
- Purslane
- Red Cabbage
- Rutabagas (Neeps Swedes)
- Savoy Cabbage
- Winter Squash
- Scallop Squash
- Snow Peas
- Spinach
- Taro
- Tomatoes
- Turnip Greens
- Turnips
- Winter Squash
- Yam
- Yellow Snap Beans
- Yellow Sweet Corn
- Zucchini
- Acorn Squash
- Alfalfa Sprouts
- Arrowhead
- Arrowroot
- Artichokes
- Arugula
- Asparagus
- Baby Carrots
- Bamboo Shoots
- Beet Greens
- Beets
- Bitter Melon
- Bok Choy
- Borage
- Broccoli
- Brussels Sprouts
- Burdock Root
- Butterhead Lettuce
- Butternut Squash
- Cabbage
- Cabbage Creamed
- Canned Asparagus
- Canned Green Beans
- Canned Mushrooms
- Canned Pimentos
- Carrots

3

Baked Foods

- Archway Home Style Cookies Sugar Free Oatmeal
- Bagel
- Basbousa
- Biscuit Cheese
- Bread Cheese
- Bread Italian
- Bread Oat Bran
- Bread Oat Bran Toasted
- Bread Oatmeal
- Bread Oatmeal Toasted
- Bread Onion
- Bread Onion Toasted
- Bread Potato
- Bread Potato Toasted
- Bread Soy
- Churros
- Cracker Meal
- Crackers Milk
- Crisp Blueberry
- Crisp Cherry
- Crisp Peach
- Crisp Rhubarb
- Dessert Pizza
- Dumpling Plain
- English Muffins
- English Muffins Mixed-Grain
- Fig Bars
- Forunte Cookies
- French Bread

- Molasses Cookies
- Oatmeal Cookies
- Pie Peach
- Pita Bread
- Roll Garlic
- Rye Bread
- Strudel Cherry
- Strudel Peach
- Strudel Pineapple
- Taco Shell Flour
- Toasted Bagels
- Turnover Guava
- Waffle Buttermilk Frozen Ready-To-Heat Toasted
- Waffles Gluten-Free Frozen Ready-To-Heat
- Wheat Bread
- White Bread
- Whole Wheat Bread
- Whole Wheat Pita

Beverages

- Aloe Vera Juice Drink Fortified With Vitamin C
- Black Tea (Brewed)
- Bottled Water
- Caffeine Free Cola
- Cantaloupe Nectar
- Cereal Beverage (non-alcoholic)
- Chicory Beverage
- Chocolate Almond Milk
- Chocolate Drink Powder
- Citrus Energy Drink
- Club Soda
- Coffee
- Coffee Turkish
- Corn Beverage (non-alcoholic)
- Cream Soda
- Decaf Coffee
- Diet Cola
- Diet Green Tea
- Energy Drink
- Espresso
- Frozen Coffee Drink
- Frozen Coffee Drink Decaffeinated
- Frozen Daiquiri
- Grape Soda
- Green Tea
- Irish Coffee
- Low Calorie Cola
- Orange Soda
- Peach Nectar
- Protein Powder Soy Based
- Tap Water
- Tea Green Brewed Decaffeinated
- Tea Green Brewed Regular
- Tea Hot Chai With Milk
- Tea Instant Lemon Diet
- Tonic Water
- Unsweetened Rice Milk
- Vitamin Fortified Water
- Water Non-Carbonated
- Well Water
- Whey Protein Powder Isolate

Dairy and Egg Products

- Almond Milk Unsweetened
- Breast Milk (Human)
- Buttermilk
- Dried Sweet Whey Powder
- Dried Whey Powder (Acid)
- Egg White Dried
- Egg White Powder
- Egg Whites
- Fat Free Cream Cheese
- Fatfree Chocolate Milk
- Goat Milk
- Greek Yogurt (Plain)
- Hot Cocoa
- Low-Fat Milk 1%
- Low-Fat Milk 2%
- Low-Fat Yogurt
- Lowfat Buttermilk
- Non-Fat Yogurt
- Plain Yogurt
- Skim Milk
- Whey Acid Fluid
- Whole Milk
- Yogurt Coconut Milk
- Yogurt Liquid

Fats and Oils

- Almond Oil
- Avocado Oil
- Canola Oil
- Cocoa Butter
- Coconut Oil
- Corn Oil
- Cottonseed Oil
- Flaxseed Oil
- Grapeseed Oil
- Hazelnut Oil
- Margarine
- Margarine (Unsalted)
- Mustard Oil
- Oil Babassu
- Oil Nutmeg Butter
- Oil Oat
- Oil Sheanut
- Olive Oil
- Palm Oil
- Peanut Oil
- Poppyseed Oil
- Rice Bran Oil
- Sesame Oil
- Sesame Seed Dressing
- Soybean Lecithin
- Soybean Oil
- Tomatoseed Oil
- Vegetable Shortening
- Walnut Oil
- Wheat Germ Oil

Sweets

- Almond Joy Candy Bar
- Baby Ruth
- Candied Tamarind
- Caramel Candy
- Caramel With Nuts
- Chewing Gum
- Cocoa Dry Powder
- Cocoa Powder
- Date Candy
- Gelatin Dessert
- Gelatin Dessert With Fruit
- Gelatin Snacks
- Guava Paste
- Halavah Plain
- Halvah Plain
- Haupia
- Honey
- Ice Creams Vanilla Fat Free
- Jellies
- Jellybeans
- Meringues
- Molasses
- Nougat Chocolate Covered
- Nougat With Almonds
- Peanut Bar
- Reeses Bites
- Sesame Crunch
- Sugar
- Sugars Maple
- Sugars Powdered
- Sweet Chocolate
- Syrup Cane
- Syrup Dietetic
- Syrups Maple
- Syrups Sorghum
- Taffy
- Toffee Plain
- Toppings Pineapple

- Toppings Stberry
- Yokan
- York Bites

Soups and Sauces

- Barbecue Sauce
- Borscht
- Cheese Dip
- Cheese Sauce
- Chutney
- Eggplant Dip
- Fish Broth
- Fish Stock
- Gravy Redeye
- Hoisin Sauce
- Hot Sauce
- Hummus Flavored
- Hummus Plain
- Instant Soup Noodle
- Manhattan Clam Chowder
- Minestrone
- Miso Sauce
- Osyter Sauce
- Pasta Sauce
- Pesto
- Pimiento
- Potato Chowder
- Recaito
- Seaweed Soup
- Soup Fruit
- Spinach Soup
- Sriracha
- Tabasco Sauce
- Tomato Relish
- Vegetable Broth
- Vegetable Soup
- Wasabi
- Worcestershire Sauce
- Yeast Extract Spread
- Zucchini Soup Cream Of Prepared With Milk

Spices and Herbs

- Anise Seeds
- Balsamic Vinegar
- Basil
- Bay Leaves
- Caay Seed
- Capers
- Cardamom
- Cayenne Pepper
- Celery Seed
- Chili Powder
- Cinnamon
- Coriander Seed
- Cumin Seed
- Curry Powder
- Dill
- Dried Basil
- Dried Chervil
- Dried Coriander
- Dried Dill Weed
- Dried Marjoram
- Dried Oregano
- Dried Parsley
- Dried Rosemary
- Dried Spearmint
- Dried Tarragon
- Fennel Seed
- Garlic Powder
- Ground Allspice
- Ground Cloves
- Ground Ginger
- Ground Mace
- Ground Mustard Seed
- Ground Nutmeg
- Ground Sage
- Ground Savory
- Ground Turmeric
- Horseradish
- Onion Powder
- Paprika
- Peppermint
- Poppy Seeds
- Rosemary
- Saffron
- Table Salt
- Thyme (Fresh)
- Vanilla Extract
- White Pepper
- Yellow Mustard

Snacks

- Bean Chips
- Corn Cakes
- Corn Chips Flavored
- Corn Chips Flavored (Fritos)
- Corn Chips Plain
- Crackers Rice And Nuts
- Popcorn
- Pretzels Soft Nfs
- Rice Crackers
- Rice Paper
- Soft Pretzels
- Soychips
- Trail Mix
- Vegetable Chips

Nuts and Seeds

- Acorns
- Almond Butter
- Almond Paste
- Almonds
- Brazilnuts
- Butternuts
- Cashews
- Chestnuts
- Chia Seeds
- Chinese Chestnuts
- Coconut Milk
- Dried Beechnuts
- Dried Chinese Chestnuts
- Dried Coconut
- Dried Coconut (Unsweetened)
- Dried Ginkgo Nuts
- Dried Hickorynuts
- Dried Japanese Chestnuts
- Dried Lotus Seeds
- Dried Pilinuts
- Dried Pine Nuts
- Dried Pumpkin And Squash Seeds
- Dried Sunflower Seeds
- Dry Roasted Almonds
- Dry Roasted Hazelnuts
- Dry Roasted Macadamia Nuts
- Dry Roasted Peanuts
- Dry Roasted Pecans
- Dry Roasted Pistachio Nuts
- Dry Roasted Sunflower Seeds
- Dry Roasted Sunflower Seeds (With Salt)
- Dry-Roasted Cashews
- Dry-Roasted Mixed Nuts (Salted)
- Flax Seeds
- Hazelnuts
- Lotus Seeds
- Macadamia Nuts
- Mixed Seeds
- Nuts Acorns
- Nuts Almond Butter Plain With Salt Added
- Pecans
- Pistachio Nuts
- Pumpkin Seeds Salted
- Safflower Seeds
- Sesame Butter (Tahini)
- Sesame Seeds
- Walnuts
  - Walnuts Honey Roasted
- Sesame Butter (Tahini

Grains and Pasta

- Amaranth
- Brown Rice
- Bulgur
- Couscous
- Millet
- Oat Bran
- Oatmeal
- Pasta (Unenriched)
- Teff
- Wild Rice
- Amaranth Grain Un
- Brown Rice
- Canned Hominy
- Congee
- Cornstarch
- Couscous Dry
- Gluten Free Corn Noodles
- Kamut
- Millet
- Millet Flour
- Oat Bran
- Pasta
- Quinoa
- Rice Bran
- Triticale
- Un Oats
- Un Whole-Grain Cornmeal
- Vital Wheat Gluten
- Wheat Durum
- Wheat Germ Crude
- Wheat Sprouted
- White Rice
- Whole Wheat Pasta
- Wild Rice

FRUITS

- Acerola Juice
- Ambrosia
- Apple Juice
- Apples
- Applesauce Canned or Unsweetened
- Apricots
- Asian Pears
- Avocados
- Bananas
- Bartlett Pears
- Blackberries
- Blueberries
- Bosc Pear
- Boysenberries
- Boysenberries Canned Heavy Syrup
- California Avocados
- California Grapefruit
- California Valencia Oranges
- Canned Orange Juice
- Cantaloupe Melons
- Carissa
- Casaba Melon
- Cauliflower Pickled
- Celery Pickled
- Cherimoya
- Cherries (Sweet)
- Clementines
- Corn Relish
- Crabapples
- Cranberries
- Dates
- Dried Apples
- Dried Apricots
- Dried Bananas
- Dried Blueberries (Sweetened)
- Dried Cranberries (Sweetened)
- Dried Figs
- Dried Jujube

- Dried Litchis
- Dried Longans
- Dried Peaches
- Dried Peaches (Low-Moisture)
- Dried Pears
- Dried Sweetened Mango
- Durian
- Elderberries
- Feijoa
- Figs
- Florida Avocados
- Florida Grapefruit
- Florida Oranges
- Frozen Raspberries
- Frozen Stberries
- Gala Apples
- Gooseberries
- Grape Juice
- Grapefruit
- Grapefruit Juice
- Grapes
- Grapes Canned
- Green Olives
- Groundcherries
- Guavas
- Jackfruit
- Kiwifruit
- Lemon Juice
- Lemon Peel
- Lemons
- Lime Juice
- Limes
- Litchis
- Longans
- Loquats
- Mangos
- Melon Balls
- Mulberries
- Mushrooms Pickled
- Navel Oranges
- Nectarines
- Oheloberries
- Olives

- Orange Juice
- Oranges
- Papaya
- Pears
- Pineapple
- Pineapple Dried
- Pitanga
- Plums
- Pomegranates
- Prune Dried With Sugar
- Prune Puree
- Prune Whip
- Prunes (Dried Plums)
- Pummelo
- Raisins
- Raspberries
- Rhubarb
- Rowal
- Soursop
- Sugar Apples
- Tamarinds
- Tangerine Juice
- Tangerines
- Turnip Pickled
- Vegetable Relish
- Watermelon
- White Grapefruit
- White Grapefruit Juice
- Yellow Peaches
- Zante Currants

Lentils and Beans

- Lupin Beans
- Miso
- Navy Beans
- Okara
- Papad
- Peanut Flour Low Fat
- Silk (Soy Milk)
- Soft Tofu
- Soy Milk
- Soy Sauce
- Split Peas
- Tamari
- Tofu Yogurt
- Unsweetened Soy Milk
- Vanilla Soy Milk
- Vegetarian Fillets
- Vegetarian Stew

- Blackeyed Peas
- Broadbeans
- Catjang Beans
- Peanuts
- Red Kidney Beans
- Adzuki Beans
- Bean Cake
- Beans Yellow Mature Seeds
- Black Beans
- Black-Eyed Peas (Cowpeas)
- California Red Kidney Beans
- Canned Baked Beans
- Canned Cranberry Beans
- Canned Kidney Beans
- Canned Navy Beans
- Chickpea Flour (Besan)
- Chickpeas Dry
- Dry-Roasted Soybeans
- Edamame
- Falafel
- Firm Tofu
- Fortified Silken Tofu
- Green Soybeans
- Kidney Beans
- Lentils
- Lima Beans
- Loaf Lentil